A PHARMACIST'S GUIDE to CANNABIS

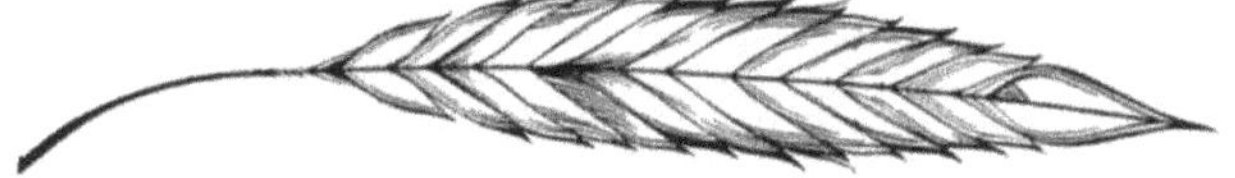

Perspective of a non-conformist clinician

Dr. Lola Ohonba, Pharm.D.

DEDICATION

This book is dedicated to our Almighty God, the creator of the universe, including botanicals such as cannabis.

I would also like to dedicate this book to the memory of my mom and dad (Martha and Julius); my boo, "Actor Charles"; and our 3 "Amigos," William, CJ, and Immanuel.

MEDICAL DISCLAIMER

This book is for educational purposes and should not be taken as medical advice. Consult with your health-care provider for all your medical needs. Do not start or stop any medication (including herbal supplements) without talking with your doctor. As at the time of publishing this book, all supplements including over-the-counter vitamins and cannabis-infused products are not FDA approved. We do not claim that supplements including cannabinoids heal, treat, or cure disease.

CONTENTS

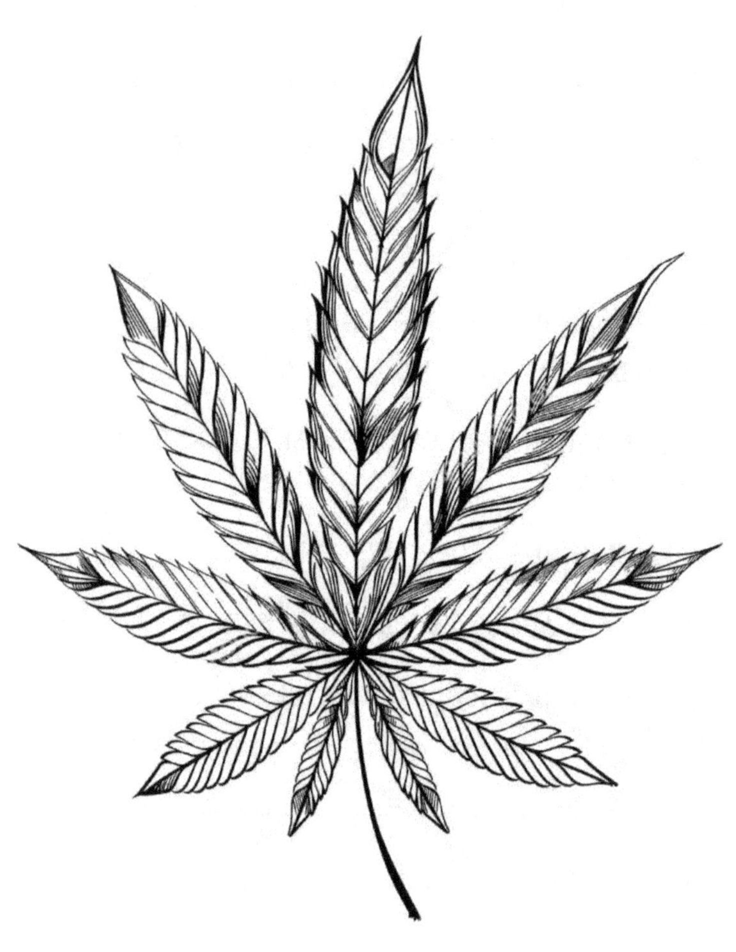

INTRODUCTION

A Pharmacist's Guide to Cannabis is written to be short, funny, and to the point for easy reading. The attempt at humor was intentional in order to remove the medical jargon often found in medically-focused books.

The legalization of both medical and recreational cannabis continues to spread not just across the country, but all over the world. As at the time of writing this book, either medical or recreational cannabis is now legal in 33 states and Washington, D.C. (approximately 170 million people living in these areas). The medical cannabis market is projected to be worth up to $11 billion in the United States in the year 2020 alone.

In its press release dated June 12, 2020, the World Health Organization (WHO) removed cannabis from the "drug" category. According to the press release, "The WHO document recognizes that there are no reported cases of abuse or dependence on the substance, and that it does not represent a danger to public health."

WHO specified that cannabidiol is not addictive; however, despite this, it does not mean that cannabis is no longer classified as a drug by international health organizations. The

WHO report only indicates the results for one of the elements of cannabis: cannabidiol (CBD).

I wrote this book to get you ready for what is to come in the cannabis space. Cannabis and other medicinal plants will be legalized whether the greedy corporations like it or not – it's just a matter of time.

The tide is changing. Countries like South Africa have already legalized not just medicinal but recreational cannabis as well. According to South Africa's Supreme Court, cannabis prohibition is a violation of its citizen's human rights.

So, where will you be when the wave comes crashing in? Are you going to sit on the sideline, and let the "wave" pass you by ...?

Or, are you going to take your health and wealth into your own hands by learning the essential facts that are going to be necessary to navigate the emerging market? Are you going to do whatever it takes to learn the basics of this amazing "wonder plant" that our creator has blessed us with richly to enjoy?

According to the biblical saying: "My people perish for lack of knowledge."

I believe nature has given unto us ALL that we need to live a healthy and sickness-free life. I believe knowledge is power. I encourage you to empower not just yourself but also your loved ones with a copy of *A PHARMACIST'S GUIDE TO CANNABIS: Perspective of a non-conformist clinician* today before the "WAVE" comes crashing in.

CANNABIS: PERSPECTIVE OF A NON-CONFORMIST CLINICIAN

Cannabis like other botanicals such as ginger, garlic, and lemongrass has been around dating back to 700 BC, and been used for the management of various disease states. In fact, cannabis might be the most versatile plant known to humankind.

As a clinician, I'm not naive enough to think there's "one miracle drug" that can cure all diseases. Cannabis is not a "wonder drug" that can cure all diseases either. But cannabinoid products have been used for generations to manage over 100 disease states including melancholy (depression).

As a clinical pharmacist, I worked directly with patients for many years in a retail setting, and later transitioned to managed care (HMO, PBM), where I still work.

It breaks my heart when a patient comes into the pharmacy with a prescription request that I know has better alternatives but I am unable to the change request to what is best for the patient, both in terms of side effects profile or cost, either due to preset formulary, bureaucracy, or corporate greed.

Why do you think "big pharma" and corporations are fighting tooth and nail to prevent the legalization of cannabis?

Why do you think they spend billions of dollars every year lobbying our lawmakers, who we sent to Washington to represent and protect us from "Sherlock Holmes" like them?

Big pharma and corporations know that the day cannabis is legalized will be the end of the feeding of their insatiable hunger for "more wealth" at the expense of poor and middle-class people like you and me.

Imagine what would happen to big pharma like Purdue, if cannabis were to be legalized today – and millions of people don't have to take their opioids for pain and die of an overdose, or suffer from drug addiction anymore.

Well, I'll tell you what would happen – they'll have to say "Bye, Felicia" to their big yacht, Swiss and offshore bank accounts, and their multi-million dollar mansions in the Islands, off my home state of Florida (i.e., Bahamas, Turks & Cacaos, and my very fave, Cayman Island – where heaven and hell still exist side by side ... lol).

I know what you guys are thinking about the Cayman part ... How did you know all that about Cayman? Did you travel down there ...? If yes, then how can you say you're not just one of the big pharma? Ha ha ...

Trust me, people, I'm not one of them at all (I'm one of the working poor actually ☹). Remember I told you guys I live in Florida? Well, here is how I made it happen:

- Florida is just a few hours from most of the Islands. It's a lot cheaper to travel to the Island via a cruise, cos I didn't have to pay extra for food, hotels, flight, or entertainment … wink wink 😊
- Finally, I'd save for a whole year just to make that trip (in fact, the proximity to most of the Islands and the opportunities to travel to that part of the world was one of my main reasons for moving to the Sunshine State in the first place, despite the fact that most of the craziest things in the world tend to happen in Florida, and the Bronx, NY 😊). Now back to reality.

Before the prohibition of 1937 and the passage of the Marihuana Tax Act, which later resulted in cannabis being federally illegal, the doctor's offices and big pharma like Eli Lily were said to have compounded cannabis tinctures and sold them as medicinal cannabis oil to people for the treatment of various illness ranging from depression, neuropathic pain, muscle spasm, and menstrual pain, just to mention a few.

I guess cannabis was the "GOLD RUSH" of their time and we definitely have to give it to big pharma to ALWAYs shows up where money is being made (I'm not mad about corporations making money. I'm a capitalist myself, but being greedy at the expense of the health and well-being of poor people is the part that leaves a bitter taste in my mouth).

Did you know that as far back as the 1900s, Queen Victoria of England was said to have used cannabis tinctures for severe menstrual pain? I would think that, what is good for the Queen, should be good for the rest of us … Just saying!

Cannabis was removed from the US Pharmacopeia in 1941. Its removal has had a wide range of negative effects on the society, resulting in the spread of outright lies and denial of its medicinal properties.

Prohibition also resulted in cannabis being classified as a Schedule 1 drug in the same class as heroin, LSD, and cocaine. Schedule 1 drugs are drugs with no accepted medical uses, high potential for abuse, and the most dangerous with potential for severe psychological or physical dependence.

If cannabis is that dangerous, why do we prescribe and dispense the single-molecule synthetic cannabinoids such as Marinol and dronabinol (without the entourage effects seen in whole plants or broad-spectrum extracts) to our most vulnerable patients as seen in cancer patients for nausea and vomiting due to chemo, or to our HIV/AIDS population for weight loss due to HIV/AIDS?

Mind you, nobody has ever died of a cannabis overdose that we know of so far ... I think it's absolutely ridiculous to have classified cannabis as the "most dangerous" drug, when according to CDC, there has been no record of cannabis-related overdose documented so far.

Evidence has shown that cannabis is less harmful than alcohol, tobacco and *way* less harmful compared to opioids such as fentanyl, OxyContin, oxycodone, and oxymorphone just to mention a few. And these opioids are classified in Schedule 2 below cannabis.

So, what happened from the time cannabis was being used for almost all ailments to it being classified as the most dangerous drug on the planet ...?

What happened, has got nothing to do with either the efficacy of the cannabis plant, the little-to-no side effects, or its so-called addictive nature.

CANNABIS PROHIBITION
IS ALL ABOUT ...

1. Antiimmigration sentiment brought about by the joblessness resulting from the great depression (kind of like the rhetoric we're hearing in our country at the moment as well).

2. The biggest reason why I think cannabis was prohibited in my opinion is the insatiable greed of big pharma and corporations.

3. The big corporations were afraid of what would happen to their bottom line if cannabis was to remain legal. So, they had to do whatever it takes to get this amazing plant out of the hands of regular folks like you and me who need it the most, including lying through their teeth.

4. That's why we need to get public funding out of polities.

Over the years, botanicals such as cannabis have been made the "bogeyman" by greedy people who only care about their bottom line. These set of people and corporations never give a damn whether you can't put food on your family's table or go bankrupt trying to pay for health care.

So many lies have been spread for so long that the average person doesn't have a choice but to believe the lies. Well, "We the people" have chosen knowledge over ignorance, and are refusing to believe in their lies anymore.

Cannabis and other botanicals are NATURAL PLANTs given to US by our maker to enjoy. Botanicals are not perfect, but the real "BAD GUYS" are the corporation feeding people "garbage" and getting them hooked up on bad drugs. Here are some of the lies that have been spread for generations about cannabis:

Myths (aka LIES) surrounding cannabis

- Cannabis leads to opioid use and abuse.
- Cannabis causes physical dependence and the experience of withdrawal.
- Over time, cannabis permanently changes brain cells and causes permanent memory loss.
- Cannabis users are less motivated and less productive compare to non-users.

Facts you should know about cannabis:

1. Pregnant women of the Rastafarian descendants of Jamaica were said to have used cannabis to control pregnancy-induced nausea and vomiting, and pain due to childbirth.

2. As a mother, I've had to use an epidural during delivery; trust me, it's not fun even with the so-called epidural.

3. Have you ever wondered how the women of old were able to go through labor without the convenience of modern medicine ...? Well, now you know!

4. Early men and women were said to have used cannabis as a tonic, which in our modern time would be equivalent to multivitamins and supplements that we now buy over the counter (OTC).

5. Marijuana and the hemp plant both belong to the cannabis family.

6. The difference between marijuana and hemp is the concentration of THC found in the flower or leaves of both plants.

7. Industrial hemp is classified as cannabis with less than or equal to 0.3% THC.

8. Due to the passage of the "Farm Bill" by United States Congress in 2018, industrial hemp-derived CBD is now federally legal to use, sell, and carry across state lines (THC < or = 0.3%).

9. Cannabis oil is low in saturated fat, which is very good for maintaining heart health, low cholesterol and reducing diabetes.

10. Cannabis and hemp products were not just used as food but also as natural fibers, used in making clothes and paper products.

11. The declaration of independence was written on hemp-derived paper.

12. The Asia of old, including the Chinese and the Indians were said to have used cannabis as medicine for various ailments.

13. According to historians, cannabis was used in the early ages to control symptoms of post-traumatic stress disorder (PTSD).

14. Cannabidiol (CBD) is the primary non-psychoactive compound in the cannabis plant.

15. Tetrahydrocannabinol (THC) is the psychoactive compound in the cannabis plant.

16. Pain is the number one medical condition why people use cannabinoid-based products, especially when traditional therapy like opioids such as fentanyl patches, OxyContin, and hydrocodone is tried and fails.

17. Cannabinoids such as THC are said to have 20 times the anti-inflammatory properties of NSAIDs (nonsteroidal anti-inflammatory drugs such as ibuprofen, naproxen, aspirin).

18. There has been no documentation of cannabis or cannabinoid-related overdose.

19. Most adverse effects of cannabinoids are minor, short term, and easily reversible after discontinuation or dose reduction of the products.

20. Studies have ranked cannabis as less addictive than cocaine.

21. Some cannabinoid compounds act in two phases (the low dose and high dose of a particular compound act in the opposite way).

22. Low dose THC tends to stimulate, while high dose sedates. When it comes to dosing of medication, including cannabinoid products, the rule of thumb is: "Start Low, Go Slow."

23. CBD has little or no known adverse effect at any dose.

24. CBD tends to reduce the negative side effects of THC, such as anxiety, short-term memory loss (among others), by reducing the binding of THC to CB1 receptors, thereby preventing THC binding.

25. Cannabinoids such as CBD and THC have the potential to treat a wide variety of health condition by directly binding and activating positive response from the receptors such as opioid, dopamine, and serotonin receptors, just to mention a few.

26. Opioid receptor – decreases pain.

27. Dopamine receptor – decreases depression.

28. Serotonin receptor – decreases anxiety.

29. Cannabinoid inhalation = rapid absorption and elimination due to no first-pass metabolism (products absorb straight into the bloodstream).

30. Cannabinoid ingestion: Effects start slow, but last longer (due to first-pass metabolism). In first-pass metabolism, drugs and food are first digested in the liver to a more active form. In the case of cannabinoid, the products are converted to a more active, longer-lasting final product.

31. THC is said to send cancerous cells into apoptosis (self-death, self-suicide).

32. Cannabinoids are said to have neuro-protective properties.

33. Studies show that cannabinoids reduced the damage to the myelin sheath caused by inflammation (neuro-protective properties [Pryce, et al., 2003]).

34. Pain is the number one medical condition people use cannabis to control, especially when traditional therapy like opioids fail.

35. THC is said to have 20 times the anti-inflammatory properties of NSAIDs (nonsteroidal anti-inflammatory drugs – ibuprofen, naproxen, aspirin), and up to 2x that of corticosteroids such as prednisone (these are the main drugs used in managing pain due to inflammation in

traditional pharmaceutics). Isn't that something ... Who knew?

36. No documentation of cannabis or cannabinoid overdose.

37. Most adverse effects of cannabinoids are minor, short term, and easily reversible after discontinuation or dose reduction of the agent.

38. Studies ranked cannabis as less addictive than cocaine (Henningfield J, Heishman S. The addictive role of nicotine in tobacco use).

39. THC and CBD are odorless.

40. Terpenes, found in aromatic oils, are also found in all botanicals and are responsible for the strong smell of cannabis.

41. States with medical marijuana legalization prescribe fewer pain killers and have fewer opioid overdoses compare to states without legalization (Colorado).

42. Evidence showed that Cannabis is more of a "route out of addiction" than a "gateway to opioid use."

43. Anecdotal observation (testimonial from users) shows that some people have been able to beat opioid addiction with the help of cannabis without the debilitating side effects commonly associated with opioid withdrawal (have to replace something with something). Marijuana has been shown to be way less harmful than opioids.

44. Cannabis does not cause physical dependence. Most Cannabis users are able to stop without adverse side effects either physical or psychological.

45. No evidence to support that cannabis kills or impairs motivation.

46. THC produces short-term memory loss, but there is no evidence to support permanent memory loss or other cognitive behavioral changes.

47. The short-term memory loss observed in THC could be harnessed to manage signs and symptoms of post-traumatic stress disorder (PTSD), especially in our military population who have had to carry and are still carrying the debilitating memory of never-ending wars.

48. No evidence to support permanent harm to the intellectual ability of cannabis users.

49. No evidence to support an increase in lung cancer due to cannabis use (potential for increase in cough, phlegm, and wheezing compared to non-cannabis user).

50. Anecdotal studies have shown that cannabis is less harmful to use compared to other alternatives.

51. Evidence has shown that cannabis is less harmful than alcohol, tobacco, and *way* less harmful compared to opioids such as fentanyl, oxymorphone, cocaine, and heroin, among others.

52. Medical studies have shown that cannabis is a neuroprotectant with potential medical benefits for many

disease states such as multiple sclerosis (MS), various types of pains, cancer, glaucoma, epilepsy/seizures, among others.

53. Endocannabinoid system (ECS) is found in the brain. The highest concentration of the ECS receptors is predominantly found in the brain.

54. The brain is already producing its own cannabis-like substances called anandamide (THC-like) and 2-AG (CBD-like).

55. If cannabis is bad for us, then how come there are ECS, anandamide, and 2-AG? Our body produces what our body needs, and finds a way to get rid of what it doesn't need.

56. Neurogenesis-neurons are produced by neural stem cells.

57. Increasing neurogenesis boosts brain functions.

58. Scientists have shown that THC can promote growth of new brain cells using the process of neurogenesis.

59. According to Dr. Xia Zhang, "Most drugs of abuse suppress neurogenesis. Only marijuana promotes neurogenesis."

60. According to Dr. Sanjay Gupta (neurosurgeon, CNN Medical Correspondent), anecdotal observation shows that "sometimes marijuana is the only thing that works."

THE ENTOURAGE EFFECTS: ONE WILL CHASE A THOUSAND, TWO WILL CHASE …?

It's true that THC and CBD are the main cannabinoids in the cannabis plant that produce its therapeutic effects. Aside from THC and CBD, there are other chemical compounds, such as cannabinoids and terpenes also found in the cannabis plant that work hand in hand with THC and CBD to give the plant its uniqueness.

The interaction of the above compounds all contribute to the therapeutic effect of cannabis and botanical generally, and the phenomenon is known as the "entourage effect." It is said that the cannabis plant contains over 400 different organic compounds that contribute to its entourage effect properties.

I normally explain the entourage effect in terms of the biblical passage (Deuteronomy 32:30), that states: "One will chase a thousand, two will chase 10,000." (I know, I know, trying to go spiritual on you guys, lol). So, if one is chasing 1,000, how many will over 400 cannabinoids, terpenes, phenols, and essential oils found in cannabis and botanical chase?

The entourage effect is one of the major reasons why single molecule pharmaceutics such as dronabinol or Marinol don't produce the exact effect seen in whole plant extracts or broad-spectrum cannabinoids.

I guess it's safe to say that the effect of cannabis or cannabinoid depends on the chemical composition of the plant or the botanical. Of all the hundreds of chemical compounds found in cannabis, at least 66 are said to be cannabinoids.

Other compounds also found in cannabis include:

- Flavonoids and phenols
- Essential oil, lipids, and waxes
- Fibers (for clothes, rope, and it's now being processed for building materials and household goods)
- Amino acids (components of organic proteins)
- Ketones (sources of energy, used in weight loss agents, ketone diets)

Studies suggest that the synergistic effects of various compounds found in cannabis help to counteract some of the perceived negative effects of cannabinoids such as THC. For example, terpene such as linalool, found predominantly in flowers, is said to reduce the anxiety induced by high THC levels. CBD is said to help counteract the irritability, short-term memory loss, and anxiety from high dose THC by adjusting the CBD:THC ratio in a compound.

THE ENDOCANNABINOID SYSTEM: ROBOCOP TO THE RESCUE

The endocannabinoid system (ECS) is a system found in all humans and some lower animals. The ECS is important to human life. Before we go on, how about we define some terms:

- Endo – means inside, within
- Phyto – plant
- Cannabinoids – some of the chemical compounds found In cannabis plants
- Phytocannabinoids – cannabinoids produced from plants (examples include CBD, THC, CBG among others)
- Endoccanabinoids – cannabinoids produced by humans and some lower animals (anandamide and 2-arachidenoylglcerol-2-AG)

Now that we're done with housekeeping, what is ECS? And what has it got to do with marijuana?

In 1964, Dr. Raphael Mechoulam, an Israeli scientist, and his research partner were credited with having isolated the two main cannabinoids found in cannabis plants (THC and CBD).

The full mechanism of how THC or CBD carries out its function in the human body was not fully understood by scientists, until 1988, when an American scientist named Dr. Allyn Howlett discovered the "endocannabinoid system."

So, what does ECS do? ECS is said to help in the maintenance of physiological balance, equilibrium in humans, and lower organisms. Back in the day, in chemistry class, we were taught that equilibrium is when the negative reaction on the left-hand side equals the positive reaction on the right-hand side. Simply put, equilibrium, or homeostasis as it is also known, is the balancing of our body's physiological processes.

According to researchers, ECS might be the most important system in the human body when it comes to maintaining health and well-being.

The ECS is said to work in the brain and central nervous system using the ligand-receptor mechanism. Ha ha ... I know what you're thinking: "Shoot me right now ... what da heck" is the ligand-receptor?

The ligand-receptor mechanism can be explained in terms of your "lock and key." The cannabinoid receptors (CB1 & CB2) are the "lock," while the ligand is the key needed to open the lock (in this case, your CBD, THC, and other chemical compounds found in the cannabis plant such as beta-caryophyllene, BCP, a terpene that's been shown to not just have terpene properties, but also acts as a cannabinoid).

The ligand generally binds to the receptors – resulting in either a chemical or physiological reaction such as calmness. This phenomenon is similar to, say, when we're coming home from work and put our house key into the lock to open the door for us to enter our home.

This phenomenon explains how cannabinoids such as THC and CBD exert their characteristic effects when consumed, the reaction or effects depends on the component of cannabinoid consumed such as terpenes, phenols, flavonoids, and strains of plant used.

For many years, nobody knew how the cannabis plant was able to have its characteristic effects on people. Scientists were aware of the fact that the human body does not produce what it doesn't need. So, how is THC, CBD, and all the other phytocannabinoids able to exact their effects on the human body? Why was ECS created if the body does not produce what it doesn't need?

Researchers have since found out that the human body also manufactures its own cannabis-like compounds (anandamide and 2-arachidonoylglcerol [2-AG]) that bind to the same receptors where CBD and THC bind to in the body ... ta-da ☺ ... Mystery solved!!!

ANANDAMIDE (Joy, Bliss)

Anandamide is similar in structure and chemical composition to THC – and produces a similar effect to THC because it predominantly binds to the CB1 receptors concentrated in the brain and CNS. Anandamide is also known as "joy or bliss" because it was found to produce a joyful response similar to the euphoria seen in THC. Anandamide, like THC, is psychoactive, and plays a major role in mood, appetite, memory, insomnia, and pain management.

2-ARACHIDONOYLGLCEROL (2-AG)

2-AG is the second endocannabinoid isolated from animals. It has similar characteristics to CBD. Like CBD, 2-AG is predominantly found in the immune cells, and also binds to CB2 receptors. 2-AG like CBD is non-psychoactive, and has anti-inflammatory properties similar to CBD.

The ECS is said to work in a retrograde fashion, unlike other systems in the body such as the sympathetic and parasympathetic nervous system (fight or flight mechanism).

Retrograde means ECS is able to carry information in the opposite direction to other body systems. By working in a retrograde fashion, ECS is able to provide instant feedback on what's going on in the body to the brain and CNS, thereby, effecting an instant response from the brain to whatever situation is going on in the body at a specific time.

I call ECS retrograde communication "title tale-telling" on other bodily systems. ECS retrograde communication is unique to this system and makes it easier for the body to respond to danger.

I think it is safe to say that the ECS is our body's foot soldier, or shall we say, gatekeeper, warning everybody of impending danger or happiness – thereby assisting the body in emergency preparedness.

Studies show that endocannabinoids such as anandamide and 2-AG are produced in the body as needed, and not stored (PRN).

If the body does not store endocannabinoids, it will make sense to use phytocannabinoids such as THC and CBD-based products as supplements when there is a deficiency in the body's endocannabinoids – or if the body is unable to synthesis its own due to a defective ECS (similar to how we isolate morphine from the opium plant and use it in pain management).

Unlike opioid addiction, where if an individual takes way more than the recommended dose of opioid, it could result in overdose, and death, studies show that there has not been any death due to cannabis overdose, because ECS is able to down-regulate the cannabis receptors.

Downregulation of the receptors is a reduction in the numbers of receptors that cannabinoids are able to bind to – especially when an individual takes way more than the recommended dose (it definitely doesn't mean you should go on a cannabis binge … Always remember: Start low, Go Slow).

Another reason why there have not been any cannabis-related overdoses is due to the fact that there are no ECS receptors in the cardiac or respiratory centers of the brain stem. The brain stem is the part of the brain that causes cardiac and respiratory depression during an opioid overdose (shuts down the heart and lung during an overdose).

The above scenario definitely makes sense, because if there are no receptors at the cardiac or respiratory center for cannabinoids to bind to, then there'll no need to shut down the heart or lung resulting in respiratory depression as seen in opioid overdose.

CANNABINOIDS RECEPTOR AGONIST

What is an AGONIST?

An agonist / partial agonist binds to a receptor and causes a specific response; for example, CBD binds to CB2 receptors resulting in an anti-inflammatory response (less pain).

Let's talk about CB1 receptor agonists

Think: Brain, CNS, spinal cord, eye, penis, vagina, ovaries, liver

TETRAHYDROCANNABINOL (THC)

- Think: Primary psychoactive CPD in cannabis, best known cannabinoid, neuroprotection

- Potential Uses: Pain reliever, anti-nausea, muscle relaxant, increase appetite, relieve pressure due to glaucoma.

CANNABINOL (CBN)

- THINK: Mild to non-psychoactivity, sedative properties

- Potential Uses: Sleep aid, pain, inflammation, antioxidant, muscle spasm (probably fibromyalgia).

TETRAHYDROCANNABIVARIN (THCV)

- THINK: Psychoactive, appetite suppressant, bone stimulant

- POTENTIAL USES: Weight loss, anti-diabetes, osteoporosis (bone loss).

TETRAHYDROCANNABINOLIC ACID (THCA)

- THINK: Natural cannabis plant, neuroprotection

- Potential Uses: Prevent cancer cell growth, osteoporosis (bone), anti-inflammatory, antibacterial agents.

Let's talk about CB2 receptor AGONISTS

CB2 Receptors

Think: Lymph, immune system, thyroid, spleen, blood, and skin

CANNABICHROMENE (CBC)

- THINK: Complex of all the cannabinoids, but potentially could be the most important. Non-psychoactive

- Potential Uses: Antibacterial, anti-inflammatory (pain), antifungal, vein relaxation, lower blood pressure, bone stimulant (osteoporosis). Isn't CBC special ...? I think so too.

CANNABIGEROL (CBG)

- THINK: "Bug killer"

- Potential Uses: Antibacterial, anti-inflammatory (pain), antifungal, lower blood pressure, prevent cancer cell growth.

FINALLY, let's bring out the "ROBO-COP" itself ... NAME IT, SHE'S GOT U ...

CANNABIDIOL (CBD)

- THINK: "SUPER CANNABINOID, non-psychoactive

Potential Uses:

1. Muscle relaxant, reduce spasms, anxiety, nausea
2. Increase appetite, pain reliever, improve sleep
3. Antioxidant, bone stimulant, anti-diabetic
4. Inhibits tumor cell growth, reduce organ rejection in transplant

5. Anti-inflammatory, prevent cardiovascular accident by reducing artery/venous blockage that could lead to heart attack or stroke

AND so much more yet to be discovered. WOW ... Isn't CBD something ...? I think so too. This is a calling for more research and declassification of ALL CANNABINOIDS and BOTANICALS from SCHEDULE 1 by the "Powers that be" ... Please declassify for the sake of our people!!!

LET'S TALK ABOUT TERPENES

WHAT ARE TERPENES?

1. More than 200,000 different compounds are found in botanicals such as garlic ginger and cannabinoids.
2. At least 200 of the compounds found in cannabis are terpenes.
3. Aromatic compounds found in ALL Plants that gives it its characteristic SMELL.
4. AROMA = FRAGRANCE, SMELL (characteristic smell of cannabis is due to terpenes).
5. Terpenes are initially said to be used by plants to protect themselves from pests and predatory animals (using their strong smell as a DETERRENT).
6. Studies have since shown that terpenes not only protect plants but also have MEDICINAL PROPERTIES that can be taken advantage of by HUMANs and other LIVING BEINGS.
7. Studies also show that up to 30% of the compounds found in SMOKED-CANNABIS are TERPENES (we'll talk about various routes of administration in upcoming episodes).
8. Terpenes help to differentiate various strains of cannabinoids.

9. Botanicals vs single molecule agents (e.g., dronabinol, Marinol).
10. BOTANICALS: active ingredients + terpenes + phenols + essential oils + flavonoids).
11. This process is called the "ENTOURAGE EFFECT" (Biblical saying 1 = 1,000, 2 = 10,000)
12. The entourage effect gives botanicals their unique properties that are hard to duplicate in labs as seen in single molecules like dronabinol – side effects unbearable for people.
13. The ratio of various terpenes in a cannabinoid gives it its POTENCY, SMELL and MEDICINAL PROPERTIES.

MYRCENE

THINK

- Mango, hops, musky odor in bay, thyme, lemongrass. Most common in cannabis.
- Mostly found in INDICA or its HYBRID STRAIN of cannabinoids.
- > 0.5% MYRCENE = INDICA = SEDATIVE PROPERTIES (couch lock syndrome).
- < 0.5% MYRCENE = SATIVA = ENERGIZING PROPERTIES.
- MYRCENE is said to act as the RAW MATERIAL for the production of other TERPENES.

MEDICINAL PROPERTIES:

- Myrcene, pinene and beta-caryophyllene combo is said to reduce anxiety.
- Combination of CBG and myrcene is said to be effective as an anti-cancer agent.
- THC and myrcene combo are said to have the potential to reduce pain, muscle spasticity, and help with sleep disorders (insomnia, sleep apnea, and narcolepsy).
- Sedative and tranquilizing properties of myrcene could have positive effects on neurological conditions such as psychosis.
- Studies show that myrcene allows large molecules (THC, CBD, etc.) to easily pass through the brain by reducing the selectivity of the "blood-brain barrier (BBB)."
- Yes, I can hear you saying … How does that affect my life?
- Our brain is a highly delicate organ, and does not allow anyone to get in willy-nilly, including some essential and life-saving drugs.
- Enhancing selectivity of the BBB helps us to get needed supplements and drugs to where they are needed in the brain (targeted therapy is the future of MEDICINE)
- NATURE's been good to US … What do you think?

POTENTIAL USES:

- Sedatives (sleep), muscle relaxants, analgesia (pain), anti-inflammatory (e.g., ibuprofen), management of neurological conditions such as epilepsy, and Parkinson's disease.
- Consumption of INDICA STRAIN of cannabinoid with MANGO could INCREASE the POTENCY of THC due to high concentration of MYRCENE in both agents.

- Myrcene is said to have a pain-relieving property similar to opioids (fentanyl, OxyContin), without the negative side effects of addiction.

LIMONENE

THINK

- Lemon, citrus fruits
- Found in large quantity in cannabis

MEDICINAL PROPERTIES:

- Improves mood
- Improves digestion
- Anti-inflammatory
- Appetite suppressant
- Studies show the ability to prevent tumor cell growth by preventing blood supply to the tumor cells (starvation mechanism)

POTENTIAL USES:

- Improves mood – Anxiety, depression, and other mental health conditions.
- Improve digestion – Helps with gastroesophageal reflux disease, ulcers, and other gastrointestinal disorders (dissolves gallstones).
- Anti-inflammatory properties – Anti-cancer agent, arthritis, pain, and other inflammatory conditions such as asthma.

- Appetite suppressant – Potential weight loss agent. The combination of limonene and THCV is said to be promising for weight loss especially in type 2 diabetes mellitus.
- Cosmetics and beauty products, cleaning agents, food industries as preservatives.

LINALOOL

THINK

- Flowers, perfume, and fragrances
- Produced in small quantity in cannabis

MEDICINAL PROPERTIES:

- Sedative
- Mood stabilizer
- Anti-inflammatory/analgesic
- Muscle relaxant
- Anticonvulsant

POTENTIAL USES:

- Sedation – Helps with sleep disorders, insomnia due to its calming properties
- Mood stabilizer – Helps with psychological and mental health disorders such as psychosis, Alzheimer's dementia, anxiety, reduces stress and depression, among others
- Anti-inflammatory/analgesic properties – Helps with various pain and inflammation-related conditions such as

cancer, athlete's faster recovery time, arthritis, among others
- Anti-convulsant – Helps with various epileptic and seizure disorders
- Muscle relaxant – Helps with various spasticity conditions such as muscle spasm
- Use in cosmetics and beauty products.

NEROLIDOL

THINK

- Flowers, lavender, citrus fruit
- Cannabis

MEDICINAL PROPERTIES:

- Anti-inflammatory
- Antifungal
- Antibacterial
- Anti-cancer
- Sedation
- Neuroprotectant

POTENTIAL USES:

- Antifungal – Helps with fungal infections such as ringworm
- Anticancer – Helps with tumors and various deadly cancers

- Anti-inflammatory properties – Used in pain and most conditions involving inflammation (it is said that most disease states are due to some form of inflammation or the other)
- Antibacterial – Helps with various infections due to bacteria, especially, the fact that many "bugs" are now drug-resistant due to the inappropriate use of antibacterial agents (would be nice to introduce new nature-friendly agents to help fight the ever-evolving "bugs")
- Neuroprotectant – Could help with neurological disorders such as Parkinson's disease
- Sedation – Sedative properties could help with sleep disorders
- Cosmetics for beauty products, and food industries as flavoring agents

GUAIOL

THINK

- Pine
- Evergreen trees of tropical regions

MEDICINAL PROPERTIES:

- Antibacterial
- Expectorant
- Anticancer
- Anti-inflammatory

POTENTIAL USES:

- Antibacterial – helps with bacterial infections
- Expectorant – Helps with cough, sore throat
- Anti-inflammatory – Inflammation-related pain such as arthritis and various sport-related injury
- Anticancer – helps with various cancer side effects
- Insecticides, disinfectants

CAMPHENE

THINK

- Wood, nutmeg, basil
- Cannabis

MEDICINAL PROPERTIES:

- Antibacterial
- Antifungal
- Lipid lowering
- Expectorant

POTENTIAL USES:

- Lipid lowering – Could be used in cholesterol-lowering agent, resulting in better management of cardiovascular disease and metabolic syndrome such as type 2 diabetes mellitus.

- Antibacterial/antifungal properties – helps with dermatological conditions such as eczema and psoriasis
- Expectorant – Helps with cough, sore throat
- Anti-inflammatory – Inflammation-related pain such as arthritis and various sport-related injury

PINENE

THINK

- Heavy pine smell
- Most common terpene not just in cannabis, but all plants

MEDICINAL PROPERTIES:

- Bronchodilator
- Anti-inflammatory
- Memory retention
- Broad-spectrum antibacterial

POTENTIAL USES:

- Bronchodilatory properties – Could be used in products for asthma and other respiratory conditions
- Anti-inflammatory – Use in various painful conditions due to inflammations, including sport injuries
- Anti-tumor – Could be used as adjuvant in the management of cancer and cancer-related symptoms (adjuvant = in addition to other therapy)
- Memory retention – Could help with attention deficit disorders (ADHD), and memory/cognitive-related

conditions such as Alzheimer's or memory loss due to aging
- Broad-spectrum antibacterial properties – Could be used in developing antibacterial agents covering the drug-resistant "superbugs" such as methicillin-resistant Staphylococcus aureus (MRSA)

TERPINOLENE (TPO)

THINK

- Turpentine, nutmeg, herbs, mint, tea tree and anise
- Not found much in cannabis
- Floral

MEDICINAL PROPERTIES

- Has no anti-inflammatory or analgesic properties, hence not ideal for pain or inflammatory conditions
- Antioxidant
- Anti-tumor (studies show a positive response in leukemia and brain cancer affecting glial cells)
- Sedation
- Antibacterial

POTENTIAL USES

- Antibacterial properties – Use in insecticides and cleaning products.
- Floral nature – Use in cosmetics and beauty products (body creams, perfumes, etc.).

- Sedative properties – Could be used in insomnia and other sleep disorders such as narcolepsy or shift-work sleep disorder (SWSD).
- Anti-tumor properties – Could be used in anti-cancer agents or as adjuvants in cancer management.
- Antioxidant properties – Reactive oxidative substance is been implicated in the aging process. Terpinolene could be used in anti-aging products.

OCIMENE

THINK

- Flowers, fruits

MEDICINAL PROPERTIES

- Anti-inflammatory
- Antifungal (candida species)
- Antiviral

POTENTIAL USES

- Anti-inflammatory properties – Could be used in pain due to inflammation such as sports injuries, osteoarthritis, premenstrual symptoms (PMS)
- Antifungal – Could be used in agents for ringworm, athlete's foot, and other candidiasis-related infections

- Antiviral properties – Has been shown to be effective in treating the SARS virus (COVID-19 virus belongs to the family of SARS)

Alpha-HUMULENE

THINK

- Hop, strong beers, earthy smell
- Found in many botanicals including cannabis
- Mostly found together with beta-caryophyllene (BCP)

MEDICINAL PROPERTIES

- Appetite suppressant
- Anti-inflammatory

POTENTIAL USES

- Appetite suppressant – Could be used in weight loss agents to help with obesity, type 2 diabetes mellitus, and other weight-related metabolic syndromes.
- Might also help with cardiovascular conditions by lowering weight, hence lowering cholesterol and cardiac-related events such as plaque build-up in vessels, which can prevent heart attacks or strokes.
- Anti-inflammatory properties – Could be used in pain due to inflammation such as sports injuries, osteoarthritis, premenstrual symptoms (PMS).
- Could be used in manufacturing healthier beverages and beer.

Beta-CARYOPHYLLENE (BCP)

THINK

- Non-conformist, unique, and in a class of its own
- Pepper, oregano, clove
- Rosemary, basil, cinnamon (spicy not just in look, but also in characteristics)

MEDICINAL PROPERTIES

- BCP is said to have both terpenoids and cannabinoid properties (isn't that something beautiful to behold ...?).
- BCP is said to bind to CB2 receptors, thereby enhancing the effects of THC and endogenous anandamide.
- Enhancement of THC/anandamide increases its effectiveness as an antidepressant, anti-anxiety, and anti-inflammatory/analgesic properties (less pain).
- Recent studies show that the CB2 receptor is may be responsible for anxiety and depression.
- Mood stabilizer (studies show BCP is effective in controlling anxiety and depression in animal models [Bahi et al.]).
- Sedative properties (helps with sleep).
- Antifungal.
- Antibacterial.
- Anti-inflammatory/analgesic properties. Studies show BCP is effective in reducing pain due to inflammation and neuropathy in animal models (first common food with such ability discovered so far).
- Studies shows that BCP prevents alcohol-induced liver injury (steatohepatitis).

- Studies shows that BCP has gastro-protective properties.

POTENTIAL USES

- Antifungal properties – Could be beneficial in fungal infection such as ringworm.
- Antibacterial properties – Could be beneficial in drug-resistance bacterial infection such as methicillin-resistant staphylococcus aureus (MRSA), among others.
- Mood stabilizing properties – Might help with conditions like depression, anxiety, and other behavioral disorders.
- Anti-inflammatory/Analgesic properties – Could be used in inflammatory and other types of pain.
- Its ability to prevent alcohol-induced liver injury (Steatohepatitis) could help with recovery from alcohol addiction.
- Studies also shows that BCP could help with various sleep disorders such as insomnia, narcolepsy, among others.
- Gastro-protection – Gastro-protective properties of BCP could be used in developing drugs that could be used in the management of gastrointestinal conditions such as ulcer and gastro-esophageal reflux disease (GERD).

CANNABINOID THERAPY: WHAT'S ROUTE GOT TO DO WITH IT?

There are so many cannabis products introduced into the market today, that it can be really confusing for users as to which one to choose. The effects of cannabis or cannabinoid depend on its route of administration and what it's being used for.

SMOKING

Smoking is the route of administration most people think about when it comes to cannabis. In smoking, dried cannabis flowers are burnt and inhaled through the lung as in a cigarette. There is potential for similar side effects seen in tobacco – such as bronchitis or lung irritation. Nevertheless, evidence shows that cannabis is less harmful when compared to opioid such as OxyContin or fentanyl patch.

In inhaled cannabis, the cannabinoids such as THC, CBD and terpenes are quickly absorbed and its effects noticed within minutes. Smoked cannabis is absorbed directly into the bloodstream without passing through the liver (no first-pass metabolism observed), but the effect does not last as long as some other available routes such as ingestion. The awareness of other routes of administration with better absorption and longer duration of action is giving cannabis users more options to consider.

VAPORIZING CONCENTRATES

Like smoking, vaping involves heating cannabis or cannabis oil. Unlike smoking, the cannabinoid is not burnt in vaping. Hence, there is less entourage effect observed in vaping compared to when cannabis is smoked in the form of a traditional cigarette. The smoke from burnt cannabis is said to be irritating to the lungs and may increase the risk of respiratory conditions unlike vaporized cannabis that is not physically burnt.

Concentrates comes in different forms such as DABs, SHATTER, WAX, BUDDER, BHO, ROSIN depending on the method of extraction and solvent used in extraction.

Cannabinoids are not water soluble. Aromatic alcohol such as ethanol and butanol are some of the solvents used in the extraction of concentrates. The longer the aromatic chain, the more effective cannabinoid concentrate is extracted – but longer chained hydrocarbons are said to be carcinogenic*. Some of the residual solvent tends to remain in the extracted concentrates depending on the extraction method. Accumulation of the residual solvent could worsen side effects that may be seen in the products being used.

Concentrate is made up of oil and terpenes in the cannabis plant. The cannabis plant can have up to 20% THC, while concentrates can have as high as 70–80% THC. Concentrate, due to its high strength, is used in chronic conditions like severe pain management or drug withdrawal. It's advisable for cannabis-naive individuals to stay away from concentrate.

The most popular concentrate is BHO (butane hash oil). The quality of concentrates being vaped is important when it comes to the benefits of vaping. The question of whether vaping is safer than smoking depends on the quality of what is being consumed. It is better to always follow the safety rule of thumb, which is start slow.

TINCTURES, SPRAY AND SUBLINGUAL

The mechanism of action for the above routes is through the oral mucosa. The product is absorbed directly into the bloodstream without passing through the liver (first-pass metabolism). Tinctures, spray or sublingual could be a better choice for individuals with liver disease.

SUPPOSITORIES

In a suppositories route of administration, cannabinoids are inserted through the anal area. The onset of action can be as fast as 15 minutes, and last up to 12 hours. Just like a tincture, spray and sublingual route of administration (ROA), suppositories do not pass through the liver. This route is potentially ideal for individuals who are unable to take an oral dosage form either due to nausea/vomiting, or an inability to swallow due to gastrointestinal disorders such as peptic ulcers or erosive esophagitis.

TOPICAL CANNABINOIDS: CREAM, SALVES, ROLL-ONS

Topical routes such as creams, salves and roll-ons are said to act on the uppermost layer of the skin. The onset of action is approximately 30 minutes. The duration of action varies, but could last up to 3 hours*. Topical cannabinoids exact their effect locally (products do not pass through the liver or bloodstream). In topical routes of administration, absorption is enhanced by the alcohol or lipid phase (ointment, gel vs cream). The number of cannabis-based products being used by an individual should be taken into consideration when dosing due to the addictive properties of cannabinoids.

Topical cannabinoids are said to have the potential to alleviate joint pain such as arthritis, muscle pain, skin conditions like eczema, psoriasis and certain forms of skin cancer*. Due to the anti-inflammatory, antibacterial, and immune-modulating properties of cannabis, topical cannabinoids are said to have the potential to help regulate immune responses in the skin, in skin burns and infection*. Topical routes of administration could be an alternative for individuals who would rather not use inhaled routes or traditional pharmaceutics.

EDIBLES

Cannabis is also consumed in edible forms such as baked goods (cookies and brownies). Cannabinoids consumed in edible form have longer onset and duration of action due to the fact that they pass through the liver and undergo first-pass metabolism. An inactive form of THC, 9 OH THC is converted to long-acting 11THC.

The edible route is potentially ideal for situations that do not requires immediate effect, but long-lasting duration of action. It can take up to 2 hours before the effect of ingestion is felt depending on the individual. People need to exercise caution when taking edible cannabinoids (just because we don't feel anything, as in the case of the inhaled route, immediately doesn't mean it's not working). The rule of thumb again is to "Start Low, Go Slow."

Cannabis-infused products should not be mixed with alcohol or other CNS stimulants because of the potential for addictive CNS stimulation, which could lead to increase in the psychoactive side effects of cannabis, especially with products high in THC.

LOCK IT UP

- Cannabis-infused products like cookies and brownies should not be left on an open shelf.
- Edible products should be clearly labeled to avoid unintentional consumption or harm (especially with cannabis-naive individuals).
- It's essential to store cannabis-infused edibles and other medications or supplements in a child-proof, original package.
- Keep cannabis-infused products out of reach of children.

Edible routes of administration might not be ideal for everybody. Individuals with history of liver disease need to be extra careful if considering this ROA. Cannabis and cannabinoids are metabolized in the liver. Metabolism of cannabis-infused products could put extra stress not just on the liver but also on the liver enzymes, which could lead to exacerbation of pre-existing liver injury.

Individuals contemplating cannabinoid therapy or any therapy at all, should consult with their primary physician before starting or stopping medications or supplements. The best practice is to follow the rule of thumb we encourage in the pharmacy profession and that has been mentioned multiple times in this book: "Start Low, Go Slow."

It has been said that cannabinoids such as CBD have little to no known side effects. The FDA had since come out with an ALERT about the potential for liver injury with CBD usage.

This is where education about how routes of administration can impact users' current disease states, the availability of the drug, and how long the drug lasts in the body.

In the case of CBD and potential liver damage, individuals with risk of acute hepatic impairment do not have to literally use edible routes of administration. Other routes such as sublingual (tincture), and suppositories do not pass through the liver (first-pass metabolism). These routes are absorbed directly into the bloodstream.

There is no drug, supplement, or botanical without some form of side effects or another. We have to address the issue of side effects by weighing the risk against the benefits of drug usage.

All drugs and botanicals, including cannabis-based supplements are not "wonder drug," without their own challenges. THC-based supplements can be particularly challenging due to their psychoactive properties and the potential for short-term memory loss. Dosing is key to addressing most of the above issues due to the biphasic nature of cannabis.

CONCLUSION

The future of management of disease states using botanicals, especially cannabis/cannabinoids therapy is promising. As a society, we're doing ourselves a disservice by not spending more time and money to fund research into this amazing plant that our maker has given to us richly to enjoy.

Health care costs are speeding out of control in our country compared to other developed countries all over the world.

Botanicals such as psilocybin, cannabis, and cannabinoid-based therapy could be the only alternative brake, that we need to apply before we totally spin off the "health-care cliff."

FURTHER READING:

1. *The Pot Book: A Complete Guide to Cannabis* by Julie Holland, MD

2. *The Cannabis Manifesto* by Steve DeAngelo

3. *Edibles: Small Bites for the Modern Cannabis Kitchen* by Stephanie Hua and Coreen Carroll

4. *Weed the People: The Future of Legal Marijuana in America* by Bruce Barcott

5. *Cannabis Pharmacy: The Practical Guide to Medical Marijuana* by Michael Backes

6. *A Woman's Guide to Cannabis* by Nikki Furrer

ABOUT THE AUTHOR

Dr. Lola Ohonba, Pharm.D.

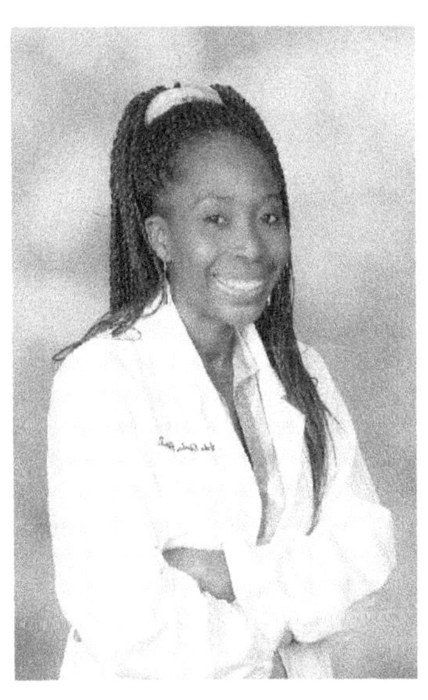

Dr. Ohonba is the founder and CEO of WCI HEALTH, an alternative health and wellness online store. She was born in West Africa (Lagos, Nigeria), and later moved to the United States. Dr. Ohonba is a clinical pharmacist certified in medical cannabis. She graduated with honors from Texas Southern University with a major in biology and a minor in chemistry. Popularly known as Dr. O, she later attended Union University College of Pharmacy in Jackson, Tennessee, where she obtained her Doctor of Pharmacy degree.

She worked for several years as a staff pharmacist for a major retail pharmacy chain (Walgreen Pharmacy). After many years of direct patient care, Dr. O transitioned to one of the top Fortune 500 companies (OptumRx – UnitedHealthcare) where she served as a clinical pharmacist in charge of prior authorization, appeals, and grievances for Medicare, Medicaid, and commercial clients. She is the host of the podcast "Let's Talk About Medical Cannabis with Dr. O" on Apple Podcast, where she talks about the role of cannabis in the management of various disease states.

Dr. O is married with three teenage boys (William, CJ, and Manny). She lives in Florida, loves to volunteer, travel, and listen to current affairs in her spare time. Dr. O is active on all social media channels. She is open to collaboration, consultation, and speaking engagements.

A MESSAGE FROM DR. O

As a clinical pharmacist, I have witnessed firsthand how patients' education and counseling have suffered recently due to unattainable goals and expectations set by big corporations for health professionals such as pharmacists. Those professionals are one of the few knowledgeable sources of truth for people to consult when it comes to clinical or nonclinical information that impacts individuals' health and well-being.

There is an opioid epidemic in our country at the moment, and the big pharmaceutical companies and corporations are the ones benefiting from it. Our people are at the receiving end of the destruction being caused by the opioid crisis.

My aim is to join all the activists who have come before me to help remove the negative stigma surrounding cannabis and other medicinal plants by providing evidence-based educational information to the general public. I believe my purpose in life is to use my God-given talent for the betterment of not just my community, but to also advance issues that affects women, children and men all over the world. At WCI Health, LLC, we provide quality products and proper health and wellness education.